I'll Do It Tomorrow

How many times have we said this?

Tidying your shed, fixing that punctured tyre or getting rid of the clothes you will never wear again.

It seems it's just too easy to watch some more TV, grab a hot or cold drink, sit and relax. That job can wait a day, then another and another.

It also seems that when it comes to our health and wellbeing we just crave another day in our comfort zone and eating that tasty sugary food. Drinking that beer or smoking that cigarette. *Just one more and then I'll quit.*

This book is advice and guidance. Take it or leave it, there is no hard sale here. I'm not affiliated to a gym or specific sport or brand. I'm just like you probably. I grew up on a poor diet supplied by my parents who knew no better and didn't have much money. I got into drinking alcohol far too early and smoked about 20 cigarettes a day from 17 until I was 32. Thinking it was cool initially and then from addiction. Then in 2012 I decided firmly to make a few changes because I was not achieving the goals I wanted. I ran regularly but also smoked. I trained with weights and kettle bell's but drank lager at the weekend. Each was cancelling out the other. I researched the internet and a few magazines. I began to train smarter, quit the cigarettes, reduced my alcohol intake to a few beers or glasses of wine once a month and changed my diet. Within a month I had lost almost a stone (6kg) and toned up.

I'm guessing by reading this, you've made a decision to change your ways a little and lose some of that body fat you're needlessly carrying around. By getting this book it shows you want to do better than you currently are. Changing your life around or just after some new advice.

We will always search for the easiest route to happiness and the "Facts" that support what we wish to hear but being in great shape and feeling good about yourself can come at a cost, a considerable one at times. You will feel pain, feel hungry and may resent the food you have to eat at times.

Running 100 metres truly as fast as you can is painful, running 200 metres at full speed is awful and sprinting 400 metres is a test of almost everything you have.

You may have to put yourself in these situations and feel that pain to better yourself depending on your goals and aims.

Fat

There is a simple equation to having low body fat:

Input – Output

If you eat 2500 calories a day but only use 2300 then those spare calories will be stored as fat.

Input

You are what you eat!

The science behind this is contradictory and can be confusing. You could consume 2500 calories worth of only potato chips, cola and butter if you so wished and you would have the energy to do 2500 calories worth of movement or simply to live.

You could consume 2500 calories of fruit, vegetables and good sources of meat and do 2500 calories of movement also.

The big question you have to ask yourself and you already know the answer to is, what effect will these foods or products have on me?

The better the food source, the better the effect it will have on your body, your muscles, organs and skin etc. If you fill your body with junk it will underperform and under recover. The better the source the better you will look, feel, perform and recover.

There are several different methods to get your nutritional requirements but these should be based around your goals of training.

Diets

Diets are what you eat and how often, the word diet is bounded around freely and for almost everything we put into our mouths, but eating is actually a lifestyle choice not a diet. You can have eating as a priority in your routine or as a second thought and make it up as you go.

There are hundreds of companies, organisations and businesses all trying to sway your opinion and get your money from you to choose their diet or book.

There is the Paleo Diet

Atkins Diet

The low Carb Diet

Vegetarian

Vegan

Grapefruit Diet

Any many, many more.

Simply, you should aim to get the best sources of food you can to support your goals. Regardless of your eating habits or diet believe it or not it **IS** much, much cheaper to eat healthily.

How much is a 1kg bag of Chocó pops against 1kg of whole oats (porridge)?

How much is an 8 pack of mini chocolate bars or potato chips vs 8 whole fresh apples or carrots?

How much is a kilo of fresh potatoes when compared to a kilo of oven fries?

How much is water from your house when compared to fizzy drinks or concentrated juices from the shop?

I could give you thousands of examples.

When I made the decision to eat and drink better my weekly food bill went down by almost 50%. In addition, my acne which I had a problem with since my teenage years vanished and I slept better not needing that 2am trip to the bathroom.

Because whole foods do not contain preservatives, added sugars and salts or other items you should not put in your body these foods are perishable. You can buy foods that are in the discount or bargain area of most supermarkets daily and with a tiny amount of work can cut, prepare and freeze them safely for use later.

Nutritious whole foods are foods that have not been tampered with or refined. Think: apples, bananas, grapes, carrots, onions, swede and cabbage etc. For meats, un-tampered with steaks, chicken breasts or legs that have not been pumped with saline or other chemical/water solutions to increase the weight.

The list of whole nutritious foods is massive so even if you're not a fan of certain types there are plenty of others to choose from. I used to hate salad and green vegetables as a child and I had to really force these foods down a few years back. Now I can't get enough of them. I love a good old big Sunday beef roast with peas, cabbage, broccoli and many other veggies. However, back to my point if you don't like one replace it with another.

Meats – Choose wisely. Butchers are better and cheaper than supermarkets and in today's day and age getting your meat off the internet from a company such as Musclefood or Live Lean (UK) is possible. They even deliver it to your door fresh.

Sugar – This is the big debate at the moment, in the 80's, 90's and naughties the whole western world was telling you to lower your fat intake, now the media has switched focus and is telling you to lower your sugar intake.

I doubt we will ever know the full truth and all sugars, same as all fats did back in the day are getting a hard time of it. The "Facts" will depend on the research you conduct. You will find the answers you want to hear by unconsciously selecting your preferences. If you want to believe sugar is better than fat and swapping your pork loin for a snickers bar you may find your journey takes longer.

I see fruit getting a hard time because it contains sugar but you need to know the difference between refined and naturally occurring sugars. The way the body's chemical compounds work with natural sugars such as fructose making whole food sugars safe to eat. Do your research on the foods you enjoy and want to eat, I could pad this book with 30 pages or more with food information but you may not like the foods I describe so it is best you research yourself. But to save your time you already know what answers you will get if you research the ingredients to a chocolate bar. When you research check your preferred foods

Glycemic Index (GI) amount or load, Wikipedia is a good place to start.

You should also keep yourself hydrated by drinking 2 - 4 litres a day of water, this does not include tea and coffee water.

<u>Deception</u>

Food manufacturers and supermarkets will try to trick people into parting with their money and openly lie and deceive you with gimmicks like low fat labels, low in sugar or carbohydrate statements. What they rarely say is what they are adding to the food to give it flavour to appeal to you. Most people shop under time pressure and don't read the labels correctly. Those that do, often don't know what to look for.

This is especially the case in fruit juices, yes they are low in fat but very excessive in sugars.   Because the fructose is removed, it's like spoon feeding yourself granulated sugar. Which will be stored as excess fat if over consumed.

Food is 'perishable,' it should stay fresh by being chilled or frozen. Manufacturers get the food most people consume to last by adding chemicals and excess salt and sugar into them.

Shakes and Potions

I'm not a fan or believer in shakes and potions, I have used them and paid for them and saw no real reward from their use. The word supplement is just that! A supplement. If you are skipping a meal a shake would be handy to give you calories. However, if you are eating correctly and getting carbs, proteins and all other nutrients from your diet and you already have a spare amount of calories in your body from excess fat then you do not need a supplement on top of it. If you are really thin or want to be the next Dorian Yates and need to gain some weight then sure, have some shakes with full fat milk.

But you also get what you pay for and many contain very suspicious ingredients and top sports personalities and professionals only get their supplements after researching in detail Informed-Sport.com because one mishap can end their career forever.

Alcohol

Most of us enjoy a beer or beverage and I still do occasionally but the truth is that they are empty calories giving no nutrition to your organs or muscles and are loaded with sugars. I was drinking with a buddy a few years ago and we were sharing a 24 pack of a certain beer. I took a few minutes to read the label on the back. Each beer was worth 274 calories and here I was drinking 12 in one sitting and eating pizza, fries, potato chips and smoking cigarettes. I was effectively self-harming and abusing my body and this is one of the moments that prompted me to act. We discussed the content and my friend said it was like eating 12 large chocolate bars. It's strange how we are happy to sit and chug beer one after the other but I doubt anyone would sit and eat 12 snickers bars one after the other.

Alcohol consumption is bad for health and fitness, you should reduce it as much as you can or remove it completely from your lifestyle until you have reached your goals.

<u>Output</u>

You need to use the fuel you put into your body or the excess will convert to spare energy for a rainy day, FAT!

You will burn a considerable amount of energy just existing, breathing, walking and sleeping even. But most people eat way more than they need, they often don't know this because even if portion sizes are small the extras in your food the manufacturers put in can seriously increase the calories you ingest.

Everyone's calorie requirement is different but an approximate value I would say is:

Men 1800-3000 and Women 1500-2500

Overweight people should stay at the lower end and those who are happy with their body image and train regularly the top end.

Your requirements also depend upon your age, lifestyle, job and training goals. Do not trust the one answer suits all solution.

If you already have excess energy (Fat) to use then you need to create a calorie deficit to tap into those reserves. If you are underweight and wish to get bigger or more muscular then you need more calories than you are currently getting and the quality needs to improve also.

<u>Training</u>

I have enjoyed several different forms of fitness and activities over the years and I am not here to promote just one. Media is full of hatred and corruption of sports, blaming certain ones for bad knees, or others for incompetent coaches etc. Some types despise each other for their variations. Such as the rivalry between Body-Building and Cross-Fit which I have never understood or wish to get into an argument about. Fitness should be enjoyable and rewarding.

I have switched how I train depending on my family circumstances, living location, free time and money available.

Sometimes I have been a member at a gym, other times I have trained by myself in my bedroom using a DVD workout such as Insanity or P90X. I have pushed myself hard with interval training on a hill side and other times enjoyed a casual 26 mile run along the coast.

Without going into to the styles and politics of each type of fitness training there are hundreds to choose from:

Weight Lifting

Resistance Training

Interval Training

Cross-fit

Insanity

T25

Jogging

Skipping

Boxing

Karate

Judo

Cycling

Skating

Skiing

Half/Full Marathons

Park-Runs

Kettle bells

Squash

Soccer

Rugby

Tennis

American Football

Boxercise

Tabatta

Spinning

Tae-Bo

Boot-Camp

Hiking

Home Training

Pilates

Yoga

All of these and many more will help you to lose fat, gain muscle, improve your wellbeing, improve your self-esteem, your breathing and your joints provided you perform correctly and rest as appropriate. Exercise combined with a healthy diet will ultimately work best for you.

If you are a bit shy or body conscious and aren't prepared to step into a gym just yet, basic equipment and body weight resistance will get you started. However you shouldn't be, many of those top gym goers started like you a few years ago.

Time

Your family routine and work load will dictate how much time you have to train and again the science behind training is varied and easily argued about. I have spent almost a full day in an ultra-event and other times when time is against me done 10 burpees with a press up every minute for ten minutes.

The excuse I don't have time is absolute rubbish. If you have time for TV, computers, facebook, twitter, news papers etc then you have time to train. 1 hour a day is under 5% of your total time, 1 hour, 5 times a week is even less.

If you can find an hour or more a day five times a week to focus on your training then great, if not, shorten the time and seriously increase the intensity.

One of my favourites is to pick four exercise such as 10 press ups, 20 crunches, 5 heaves and 15 squats and just go as fast and hard as I can round after round for 5, 10, 15, 20 or even 30 minutes depending upon the time available. Using a push, pull, core and legs exercise. You can change the exercise or amounts to suit your needs. Cross-fit uses this type of work out regularly. You can search online easily for Cross-Fit bodyweight routines.

I often see how many exercises I can do during TV adverts or as the kettle boils. Filling my 1.8ltr kettle to max and doing a plank as it heats up making use of what I call 'Idle time.'

Equipment

Gyms will usually be well stocked with state of the art equipment for you to use to train safely. Staff should give you an induction to show you the safe practices for each piece.

Training at home or outdoors with bodyweight can achieve great results and basic equipment to use at home can be found online or in the high street also. Press up bars, pull up bars or door frame hooks for sit ups etc are cheap and useful. Even a suspension trainer can be found for a reasonably low price on EBay or Amazon.

Now this is where you would normally find 50 pages of a muscle guy in each stage of a movement such as a press up or squat looking buff and in perfect positions and not out of breath.

Unless you have lived under a rock all your life you will know what exercises are so I am not going to pad the book out (making it more expensive) with pictures and condescending explanations.

Here is a list of exercises you can incorporate into your routine using just bodyweight or portable weights or Kettle Bell:

Press Ups

Wide Arm Press Ups

Close Grip Press ups

Chin Ups

Pull Ups

Air Squats

Toe/Calf Raises

Star Jumps

Mountain Climbers

Sit Ups

Half Sits

Plank

Side Plank

Crunches

Russian Twists

Bicep Curls

Bench Press

Incline Flys

Bent Over Rows

Dead Lifts

Shoulder Press

Leg Extensions

Turkish Get Up

Reverse Crunch

Tricep Extension

Snatch

Roll Out

Upright Row

Hip Extension

Wrist Curl

Burpee

Box Jumps

Kettle Bell Swings

Double Unders

Bicycles

Wall Sits

Step Ups

All I ask is whatever movements you do decide to perform you do safely and after a bit of research.

The Trap

The trap I have seen many caught in over the years and I confess I have sat in this category myself a few years back is when you are simply going through the motions of training. Driving to the gym to sit on a cycle to watch the music videos on the screen or reading a magazine. Going out for an "Intense run" but really I ended up jogging along comfortably.

Ruining my efforts by telling myself I had earned a reward or treat. Burning off 300 calories on the rowing machine and replacing them almost instantly with a cream cake or can of sugary fizzy stuff with lunch.

Beware of such traps, when you train it should be tough or at least beyond your comfort zone, keep records and push for progress constantly and keep the treats sparse. It's acceptable to have a few treats now and then but as a personal trainer friend of mine advised me, no treats until you are where you want to be at, each treat will set you back a step towards your goals.

I also recommend rare treat meals or snacks as opposed to *treat days* if you are going to treat yourself. A cheat or treat day can put thousands of un-required calories into your body which you will have to work off later. I personally allow myself 3 treats of no more than 300 calories spread through the week and only because now I'm where I want to be. My treats are not excessive, a slice of cheesecake or bar of dark chocolate or a shot of whisky. Not a whole cake or case of red wine.

1lb of body fat will fuel you for approximately 3000 calories. Please bear that in mind because if you have a stone (14lb) or more to shift your results will take time. Lack of quick results is a major factor is people quitting training and returning to their old unhealthy ways. Be patient and keep going. For those of you who want to give up cigarettes, I found it took almost six months for my breathing to sort itself out to a reasonable level to run longer than a few miles. Be patient, it took years to get unfit, it may take years to undo the damage.

Losing 1-1.5lb of fat a week is the average loss but more can be achieved if you train and eat well.

<u>Scales</u>

Scales are used to tell you how heavy you are in pounds or kilograms. Some will tell you your Body Fat content, water content and more. If you are going to use scales I urge you to do so with a bit of caution. I believe in 'Look Good Feel Good' and base my happiness on what I see in the mirror, not what I weigh.

However, scales can give you an indication of your start point and help you set yourself a target of how much weight to lose or gain. Try to avoid the temptation to weigh yourself every day or at different times through the day.

Your weight will change after meals, drinks, toilet visits etc so the information can get frustrating if you over check.

I have also found the versions that give you a Body Fat reading are unreliable.

If you can see your abs and veins in your arms then you have low Body Fat.

I apologise if this Book did not provide you with the miracle formula for losing 10lb a week or the secrets to the sofa workout. You get nothing for nothing and to get the body you want you will have to work hard and make a few sacrifices. If time is tight you may have to give up your TV or social media time, lunch hour or get up an hour earlier and train before work.

A journey of a thousand miles begins with one step, maybe reading this book was your first step to progress and I truly hope you get the body you wish for and I thank you for reading.

Don't leave it till tomorrow, make a change today.

Work Hard

Stay Strong

Peter Chaser

www.ingramcontent.com/pod-product-compliance
Lightning Source LLC
Chambersburg PA
CBHW072016280526
45788CB00005B/2066